Normal Labor

Mechanism and Management

Akmal El-Mazny

ISBN-13: 978-1514718902
ISBN-10: 1514718901

CONTENTS

INTRODUCTION

Labor is the physiological process by which a fetus is expelled from the uterus to the outside world.

The World Health Organization (WHO) defines normal birth as: spontaneous in onset, low-risk at the start of labor and remaining so throughout labor and delivery, the infant is born spontaneously in the vertex position between 37 and 42 completed weeks of pregnancy, and after birth, mother and infant are in good condition.

The three main factors which affect the mechanics of active labor are the power (uterine contractions or maternal expulsive forces), the passage (pelvis or soft tissues), and the passenger (the fetus).

Labor is divided into three main stages that delineate milestones in a continuous process: the first stage (cervical dilation), the second stage (delivery of the fetus), and the third stage (delivery of the placenta).

This book provides a comprehensive review of normal labor along with its mechanism and management, which will be of immense value for obstetricians and allied health professionals.

ANATOMY OF FEMALE PELVIS

The female bony pelvis is divided into:

– False pelvis (above the pelvic brim)

   Has no obstetric importance.

– True pelvis (below the pelvic brim)

   Related to the child-birth.

   Composed of inlet, cavity, and outlet.

Pelvic Inlet (Brim)

Boundaries

– Sacral promontory

– Alae of the sacrum

– Sacroiliac joints

– Iliopectineal lines

– Iliopectineal eminencies

– Upper border of the superior pubic rami

– Pubic tubercles

– Pubic crests

– Upper border of symphysis pubis

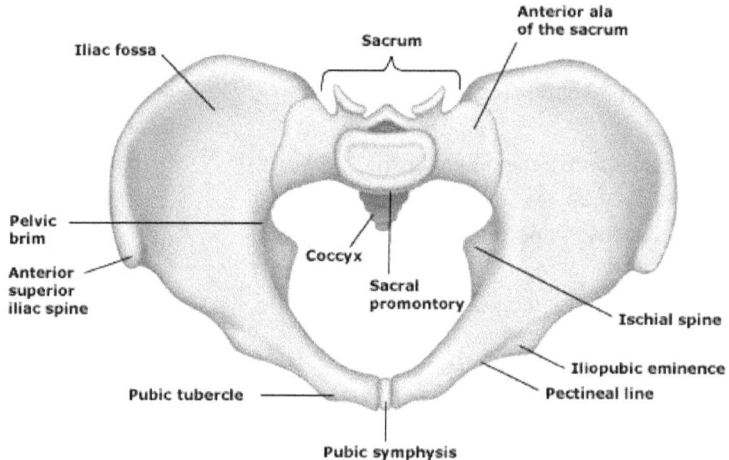

Pelvic Inlet

Diameters

Antero-Posterior Diameters

Anatomical Antero-Posterior Diameter = True Conjugate (11 cm)

From the tip of the sacral promontory to the upper border of the symphysis pubis.

Obstetric Conjugate (10.5 cm)

From the tip of the sacral promontory to the most bulging point on the back of symphysis pubis which is about 1 cm below its upper border.

It is the shortest antero-posterior diameter.

Diagonal Conjugate (12.5 cm)

From the tip of sacral promontory to lower border of symphysis pubis.

Can be measured by vaginal examination.

External Conjugate (20 cm)

From the depression below last lumbar spine to the upper anterior margin of symphysis pubis measured from outside by the pelvimeter.

It has not a true obstetric importance.

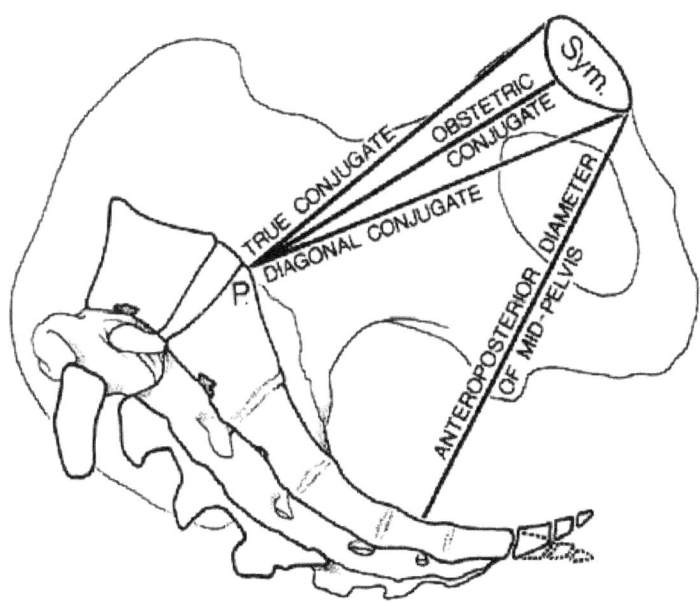

Antero-Posterior Diameters

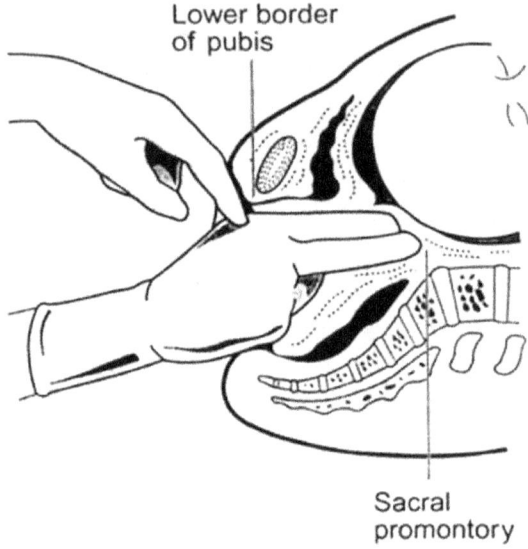

Lower border
of pubis

Sacral
promontory

Diagonal Conjugate

Transverse Diameters

Anatomical Transverse Diameter (13 cm)

Between the farthest two points on the iliopectineal lines.

It lies 4 cm anterior to the promontory and 7 cm behind the symphysis.

It is the largest diameter in the pelvis.

Obstetric Transverse Diameter (11-12 cm)

It bisects the true conjugate and is slightly shorter than the anatomical transverse diameter.

Oblique Diameters

Right Oblique Diameter (12 cm)

From the right sacroiliac joint to the left iliopectineal eminence.

Left Oblique Diameter (12 cm)

From the left sacroiliac joint to the right iliopectineal eminence.

Sacro-Cotyloid Diameters (9-9.5 cm)

From promontory of the sacrum to right and left iliopectineal eminence.

Pelvic Cavity

The roof is the plane of pelvic brim.

The floor is the plane of least pelvic dimension.

Pelvic Outlet

Anatomical Outlet

It is lozenge-shaped bounded by:

– Lower border of symphysis pubis

– Pubic arch

– Ischial tuberosities

– Sacrotuberous and sacrospinous ligaments

– Tip of the coccyx

Obstetric Outlet

It is a segment, the boundaries of which are:

- The roof: the plane of least pelvic dimension.

- The floor: the anatomical outlet.

- Anteriorly: the lower border of symphysis pubis.

- Posteriorly: the coccyx.

- Laterally: the ischial spines.

Diameters of Pelvic Outlet

Antero-Posterior Diameters

Anatomical Antero-Posterior Diameter (11cm)

From the tip of the coccyx to the lower border of symphysis pubis.

Obstetric Antero-Posterior Diameter (13 cm)

From the tip of the sacrum to the lower border of symphysis pubis as the coccyx moves backwards during the second stage of labor.

Transverse Diameters

Bituberous Diameter (11 cm)

Between the inner aspects of the ischial tuberosities.

Bispinous Diameter (10.5 cm)

Between the tips of ischial spines.

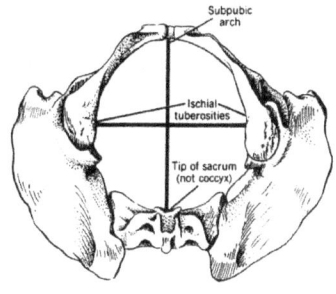
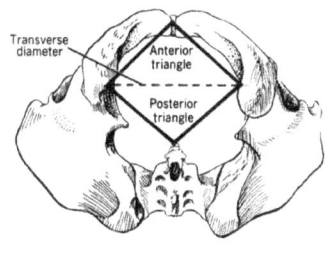

Pelvic Outlet

Pelvic Planes

These are imaginary planes lie as follow:

Plane of Pelvic Inlet

Passing with the boundaries of pelvic brim and making an angle of 55° with the horizon (angle of pelvic inclination).

Plane of Mid-Cavity = Plane of Greatest Pelvic Dimensions

Passes between the middle of the posterior surface of the symphysis pubis and the junction between 2nd and 3rd sacral vertebrae.

It is a round plane with diameter of 12.5 cm.

It is the widest part of the pelvic cavity.

Internal rotation of the head occurs when the biparietal diameter occupies this wide pelvic plane.

Plane of Obstetric Outlet = Plane of Least Pelvic Dimensions

Passes from the lower border of the symphysis pubis anteriorly, to the ischial spines laterally, to the tip of the sacrum posteriorly.

Plane of Anatomical Outlet

Passes with the boundaries of anatomical outlet.

Consists of 2 triangular planes with one base (the bituberous diameter):

– Anterior sagittal plane: Its apex at the lower border of symphysis pubis.

– Posterior sagittal plane: Its apex at the tip of the coccyx.

Anterior Sagittal Diameter (6-7 cm)

From the lower border of the symphysis pubis to the centre of the bituberous diameter.

Posterior Sagittal Diameter (7.5-10 cm)

From the tip of the sacrum to the centre of the bituberous diameter.

Types of Female Pelvis

– Gynecoid pelvis (50%): It is the normal female type.

– Anthropoid pelvis (25%): It is ape-like type.

– Android pelvis (20%): It is a male type.

– Platypelloid pelvis (5%): It is a flat female type.

– Mixed type (intermediates).

	Gynecoid	Anthropoid	Android	Platypelloid
Pelvic inlet Transverse diameter		Narrow		
AP diameter		Wide		Narrow
Forepelvis	Wide	Divergent	Narrow	Straight
Pelvic midcavity Side walls	Straight	Narrow	Convergent	Wide
Inclination of sacrum		Wide	Forward	Narrow
Pelvic outlet Subpubic arch	Wide		Narrow	Wide

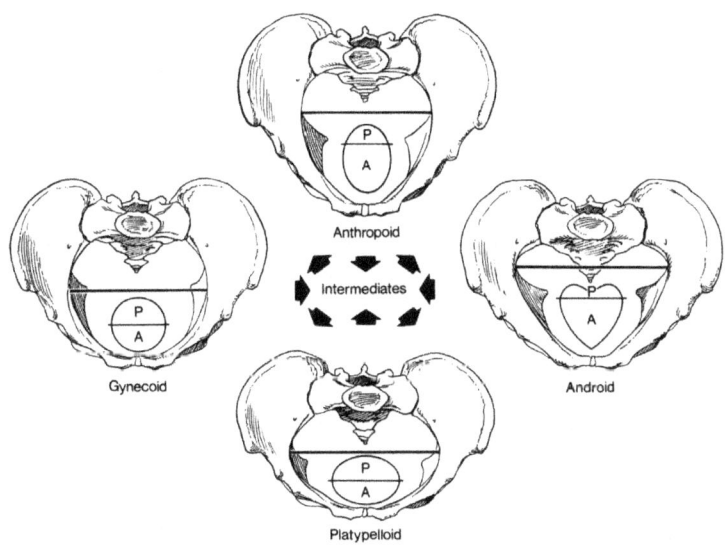

Types of Female Pelvis

ANATOMY OF FETAL SKULL

Fetal skull consists of 3 parts separated by sutures and fontanelles:

−Base: from the chin to the foramen magnum.

−Face: from the chin to the root of the nose and supraorbital margins.

−Vault: consists of three regions:

Brow

From the root of the nose and supraorbital margins to the anterior fontanelle (bregma) and coronal sutures.

It includes the 2 frontal bones separated by the frontal suture.

Vertex

From the bregma and coronal sutures to the posterior fontanelle and lambdoid suture.

It consists of 2 parietal bones separated by the sagittal suture.

It is bounded laterally by the parietal eminences.

Occiput

From the posterior fontanelle and lambdoid suture to the foramen magnum.

Sutures

Frontal, sagittal, coronal, lambdoid and temporal sutures.

Fontanelles

Four fontanelles lie at the anterior and posterior end of the temporal sutures on each side, and have no obstetric importance.

The anterior and posterior fontanelles are important to diagnose:

– Vertex presentation.

– Position of the occiput.

– Degree of flexion of the head.

Anterior Fontanelle (Bregma)

– Large, and lozenge-shaped.

– Its floor is membranous.

– Surrounded by 4 bons (2 frontal and 2 parietal).

– The floor is completely ossified 1.5 years after birth.

– The surrounding bones are not overlapping during moulding.

Posterior Fontanelle (Lambda)

– Small and triangular.

– Its floor is bony.

– Surrounded by 3 bones (2 parietal and occipital).

– The floor is completely ossified at full term.

– The surrounding bones are overlapping during moulding.

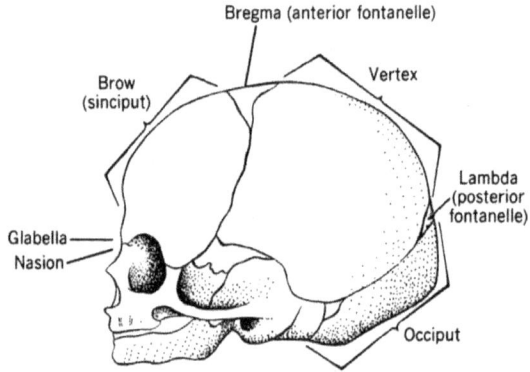

Anatomy of Fetal Skull

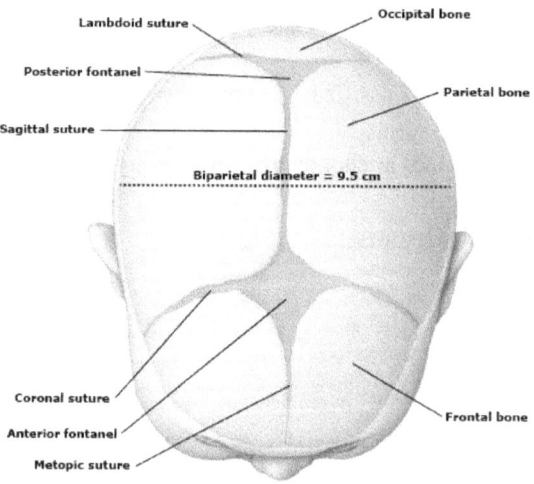

Sutures and Fontanelles

Diameters of Fetal Skull

Longitudinal Diameters

Suboccipito-Bregmatic (9.5 cm)

From below the occipital protuberance to the centre of bregma.

It is the engagement diameter in occipito-anterior with complete flexion.

Suboccipito-Frontal (10 cm)

From below the occipital protuberance to the anterior end of the bregma.

It is the diameter that distends the vulva in occipito anterior.

Occipito-Frontal (11.5 cm)

Form the occipital protuberance to the root of the nose.

It is the engagement diameter in occipito-posterior position.

It is the diameter that distends the vulva in face to pubis delivery.

Submento-Bregmatic (9.5 cm)

From the junction of the chin and neck to the centre of the bregma.

It is the engagement diameter in face presentation.

Submento-Vertical (11.5 cm)

From the junction of the chin and neck to the vertical point which is a point midway between anterior and posterior fontanelles.

It is the diameter that distends the vulva during face delivery.

Mento-Vertical (13.5 cm)

From the tip of the chin to the vertical point.

It is the engagement diameter when the head is partially extended (Brow presentation).

As it is longer than the largest diameter of the pelvic brim, the head cannot enter the pelvis.

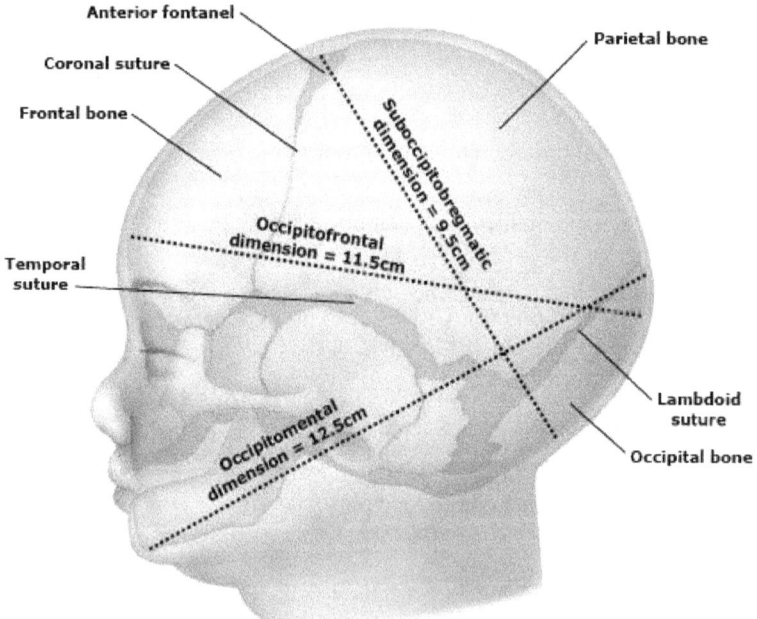

Longitudinal Diameters

Transverse Diameters

Biparietal Diameter (9.5 cm)

Between the 2 parietal eminencies.

Subparietal Supraparietal Diameter (9 cm)

From below one parietal eminence to above the opposite eminence.

Bitemporal Diameter (8 cm)

Between the anterior ends of the temporal sutures.

Bimastoid Diameter (7.5 cm)

Between the tips of the 2 mastoid processes.

Obstetric Terms

Presentation

The part of the fetus related to the pelvic brim and first felt during vaginal examination.

−Cephalic (96%)

Vertex: when the head is flexed.

Face: when the head is extended.

Brow: when it is midway between flexion and extension.

– Breech (3.5%)

– Shoulder (0.5%)

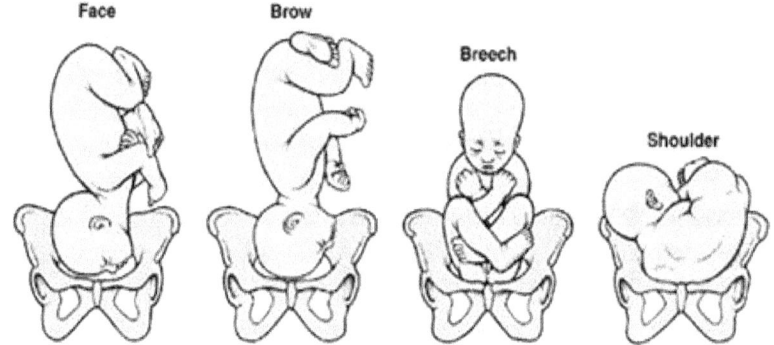

Abnormal Presentations

Cephalic presentation is the commonest as this makes the fetus more adapted to the pyriform-shaped uterus with the larger buttock in the wider fundus and the smaller head in the narrower lower part of the uterus.

Position

The relation of the fetal back to the right or left side of the mother and whether it is directed anteriorly or posteriorly.

The denominator: is a bony landmark on the presenting part used to denote the position.

– In vertex it is the occiput.

– In face it is the mentum (chin).

– In breech it is the sacrum.

– In shoulder it is the scapula.

In each presentation, except the shoulder, there are 8 positions.

In vertex presentation they are:

– Left occipito -anterior (LOA) = 60%

– Right occipito-anterior (ROA) = 20%

– Right occipito posterior (ROP) = 15%

– Left occipito-posterior (LOP)

– Left occipito-transverse (LOT)

– Right occipito transverse (ROT)

– Direct occipito -anterior (DOA)

– Direct occipito-posterior (DOP)

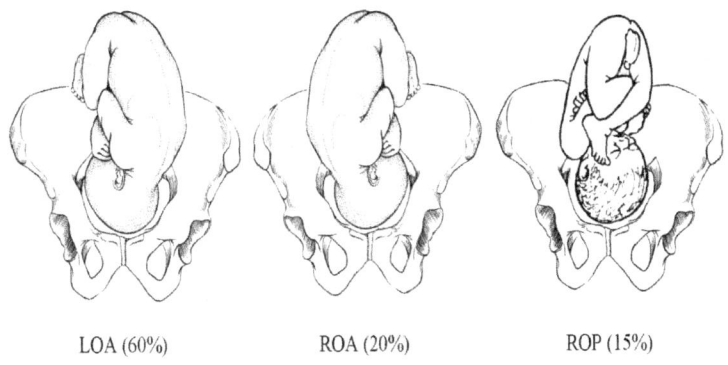

LOA (60%)   ROA (20%)   ROP (15%)

Vertex Presentation

OA positions are more common than OP positions because in OA positions the concavity of the anterior aspect of the fetus due to its flexion fits with the convexity of the vertebral column of the mother due to its lumbar lordosis.

LOA is more common than ROA, and ROP is more common than LOP as in LOA and ROP the head enters the pelvis in the right oblique diameter which is more favourable than the left oblique because:

- Anatomically, the right oblique is slightly longer than the left.

- The pelvic colon reduces the length of the left oblique.

Station

- Station 0 the vertex at the level of ischial spines (engagement).

- Station -1, -2 and -3 represent 1, 2 and 3 cm respectively above the level of ischial spines.

- Station +1, +2 and +3 represent 1, 2 and 3 cm respectively below the level of ischial spines.

Engagement

It is the passage of the widest transverse diameter of the presenting part, which is the biparietal in vertex presentation, through the pelvic inlet.

The engaged head cannot be easily grasped by the first pelvic grip, but it can be palpated by the second pelvic grip; 2/5 or less of the fetal head is felt above the symphysis pubis.

Vaginally, the vertex is felt at or below the level of ischial spines.

In Primigravida

Engagement of the head occurs in the last 3-4 weeks of pregnancy due to the tonicity of the abdominal and uterine muscles.

In Multipara

The head is usually engaged at the onset of labor or even at the beginning of the second stage due to less tonicity.

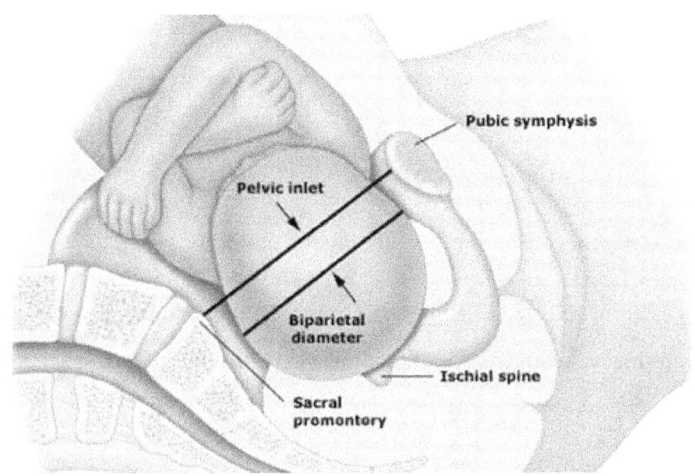

Engagement of Fetal Head

DEFINITION AND STAGES OF LABOR

Labor is the physiological process by which a fetus is expelled from the uterus to the outside world.

Delivery means actual birth of the fetus.

The World Health Organization (WHO) defines normal birth as:

– Spontaneous in onset.

– Low-risk at the start of labor and remaining so throughout labor and delivery.

– The infant is born spontaneously in the vertex position between 37 and 42 completed weeks of pregnancy.

– After birth, mother and infant are in good condition.

Labor is achieved with changes in the biochemical connective tissue and with gradual effacement and dilatation of the uterine cervix as a result of uterine contractions of sufficient frequency, intensity, and duration.

The three main factors which affect the mechanics of active labor are the power, the passage, and the passenger.

The onset of labor is defined as regular, painful uterine contractions resulting in progressive cervical effacement and dilatation.

Labor is divided into three main stages that delineate milestones in a continuous process: the first stage (cervical dilation), the second stage (delivery of the fetus), and the third stage (delivery of the placenta).

First Stage of Labor

The first stage begins with regular uterine contractions and ends with complete cervical dilatation at 10 cm.

In Friedman's landmark studies of 500 nulliparas, he subdivided the first stage into an early latent phase and an ensuing active phase.

The latent phase begins with mild, irregular uterine contractions that soften and shorten the cervix.

The contractions become progressively more rhythmic and stronger.

This is followed by the active phase of labor, which usually begins at about 3-4 cm of cervical dilation and is characterized by rapid cervical dilation and descent of the presenting fetal part.

According to Friedman, the active phase is further divided into an acceleration phase, a phase of maximum slope, and a deceleration phase.

Characteristics of the average cervical dilatation curve are known as the Friedman labor curve, and a series of definitions of labor protraction and arrest were subsequently established.

However, subsequent data of modern obstetric population suggest that the rate of cervical dilatation is slower and the progression of labor may be significantly different from that suggested by the Friedman labor curve.

Second Stage of Labor

The second stage begins with complete cervical dilatation and ends with the delivery of the fetus.

The ACOG has suggested that a prolonged second stage of labor should be considered when the second stage exceeds 3 hours with regional anesthesia or 2 hours in the absence of regional anesthesia for nulliparas.

In multiparous women, such a diagnosis can be made if the second stage of labor exceeds 2 hours with regional anesthesia or 1 hour without it.

Maternal risk factors associated with a prolonged second stage include nulliparity, increasing maternal weight and/or weight gain, use of regional anesthesia, induction of labor, fetal occiput in a posterior or transverse position, and increased birthweight.

Studies performed to examine perinatal outcomes with a prolonged second stage of labor revealed increased risks of operative deliveries and maternal morbidities but no differences in neonatal outcomes.

Third Stage of Labor

The third stage of labor is defined by the time period between the delivery of the fetus and the delivery of the placenta and membranes.

During this period, uterine contraction decreases basal blood flow, which results in thickening and reduction in the surface area of the myometrium underlying the placenta with subsequent detachment of the placenta.

Although delivery of the placenta often requires less than 10 minutes, the duration of the third stage of labor may last as long as 30 minutes.

The third stage of labor is considered prolonged after 30 minutes, and active intervention, such as manual extraction of the placenta, is commonly considered.

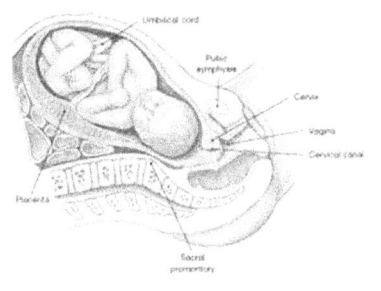

Pre-Labor

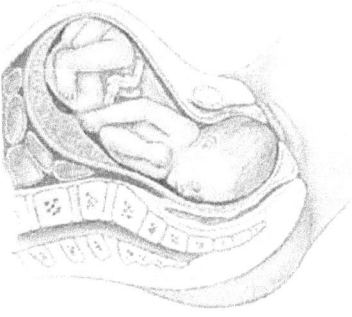

First Stage

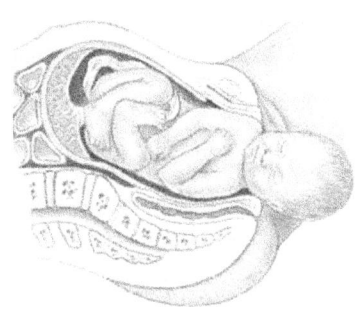

Second Stage

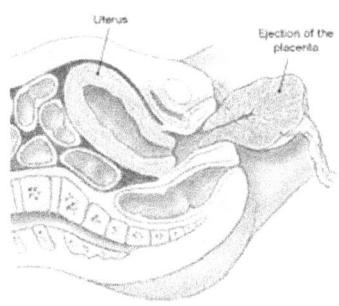

Third Stage

Stages of Labor

FIRST STAGE OF LABOR

It is the stage of cervical dilatation.

Starts with the onset of true labor pain.

Ends with full dilatation of the cervix i.e. 10 cm in diameter.

It takes about 10-14 hours in primigravida and about 6-8 hours in multipara.

MECHANISM

Causes of Onset of Labor

It is unknown but the following theories were postulated:

Prostaglandins Theory

Prostaglandins E2 and F2α are powerful stimulators of uterine muscle activity.

PGF2α was found to be increased in maternal and fetal blood as well as the amniotic fluid late in pregnancy and during labor.

Oxytocin Theory

Although oxytocin is a powerful stimulator of uterine contraction, its natural role in onset of labor is doubtful.

The secretion of oxytocinase enzyme from the placenta is decreased near term due to placental ischaemia leading to predominance of oxytocin action.

Estrogen Theory

During pregnancy, most of the estrogens are present in a binding form.

During the last trimester, more free estrogen appears increasing the excitability of the myometrium and prostaglandins synthesis.

Progesterone Withdrawal Theory

Before labor, there is a drop in progesterone synthesis leading to predominance of the excitatory action of estrogens.

Fetal Cortisol Theory

Increased cortisol production from the fetal adrenal gland before labor may influence its onset by increasing estrogen production from the placenta.

Anencephaly is associated with post-term pregnancy due to cortisol deficiency caused by lack of ACTH due to aplasia of the pituitary gland.

Uterine Distension Theory

Like any hollow organ in the body, when the uterus in distended to a certain limit, it starts to contract to evacuate its contents.

This explains the preterm labor in case of multiple pregnancy and polyhydramnios.

Stretch of the Lower Uterine Segment

Stretch of the lower uterine segment by the presenting part near term leads to reflex contraction of uterine muscle.

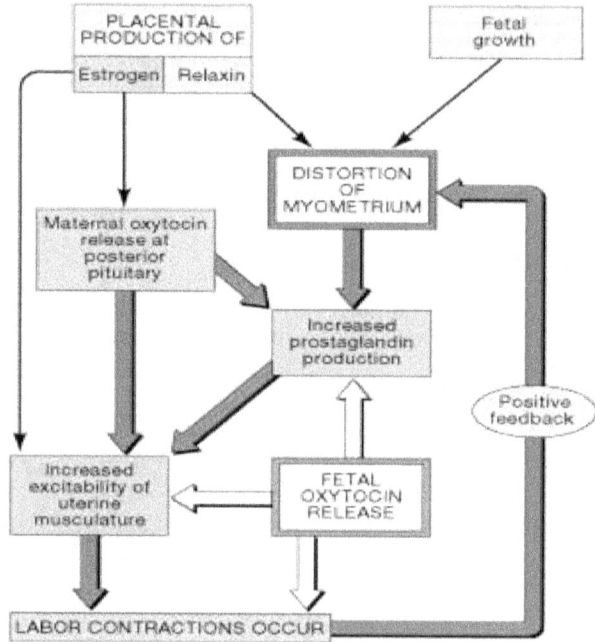

Causes of Onset of Labor

Causes of Cervical Dilatation

– Contraction and retraction of uterine musculature.

– Softness of the cervix which has occurred during pregnancy facilitates dilatation and effacement of the cervix.

– Mechanical pressure by the forebag of waters, if membranes still intact, or the presenting part, if they had ruptured; this in turn will release more prostaglandins which stimulate uterine contractions and cervical dilatation and effacement.

Mechanism of Cervical Dilatation

<u>In Primigravida</u>

The cervical canal dilates from above downwards i.e. from the internal os downwards to the external os, so its length shorts gradually to a thin rim of few millimetres continuous with the lower uterine segment.

This process is called effacement and expressed in percentage so when we say effacement is 50% it means that 50% of the cervical canal has been taken up.

Dilatation of the cervix (external os) starts after complete effacement of the cervix.

<u>In Multipara</u>

Effacement and dilatation occur simultaneously.

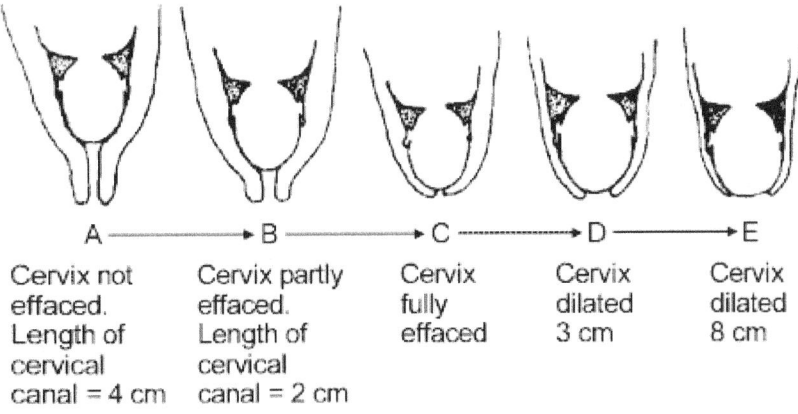

A → B → C → D → E

| Cervix not effaced. Length of cervical canal = 4 cm | Cervix partly effaced. Length of cervical canal = 2 cm | Cervix fully effaced | Cervix dilated 3 cm | Cervix dilated 8 cm |

Effacement and Dilatation of the Cervix

Phases of Cervical Dilatation

Latent Phase

This is the first 3 cm of cervical dilatation which is slow takes about 8 hours in nulliparae and 4 hours in multiparae.

Active phase

– Acceleration phase

– Maximum slope phase

– Deceleration phase

The normal rate of cervical dilatation in active phase is 1.2 cm / hour in primigravida and 1.5 cm / hour in multipara.

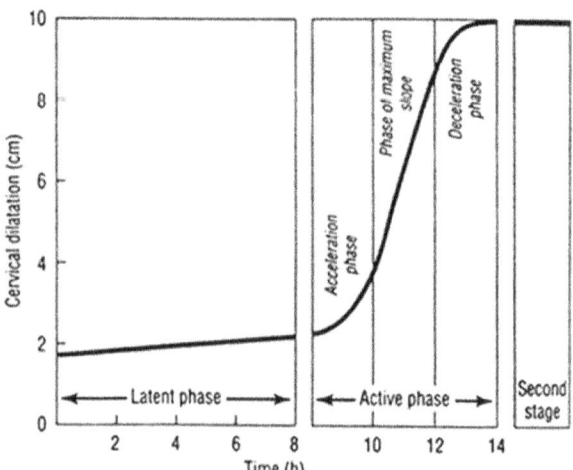

Friedman Labor Curve

MANAGEMENT

Prodromal Stage

The following clinical manifestations may occur in the last weeks of pregnancy:

Shelfing

It is falling forwards of the uterine fundus making the upper abdomen looks like a shelf during standing position.

This is due to engagement of the head which brings the fetus perpendicular to the pelvic inlet in the direction of pelvic axis.

Lightening

It is the relief of upper abdominal pressure symptoms as dyspnoea, dyspepsia and palpitation due to:

- Descent in the fundal level after engagement of the head.

- Shelfing of the uterus.

Pelvic Pressure Symptoms

With engagement of the presenting part the following symptoms may occur:

- Frequency of micturition.

- Rectal tenesmus.

- Difficulty in walking.

<u>False Labor Pain (Braxton-Hicks Contractions)</u>

These are differentiated from true labor pain as follow:

- Pain is felt mainly in the abdomen.

- Irregular.

- No increase in frequency, duration and intensity.

- No effect on the cervix.

- No bulging of the membranes.

- Can be relieved by antispasmodics and sedatives.

Onset of Labor

The onset of labor is characterised by:

<u>True Labor Pain</u>

These are differentiated from false labor pain as follow:

- Pain is felt in the abdomen and radiating to the back.

- Regular.

- Progressive increase in frequency, duration and intensity (3 contractions every 10 minutes, each lasts 50-60 seconds in active phase).

- Progressive dilatation and effacement of the cervix.

- Membranes are bulging during contractions.

- Not relieved by antispasmodics or sedatives.

The Show

It is an expelled cervical mucus plug tinged with blood from ruptured small vessels as a result of separation of the membranes from the lower uterine segment.

Labor usually starts several hours to few days after show.

Dilatation of the Cervix

A closed cervix is a reliable sign that labor has not begun.

In multigravida the cervix may admit the tip of the finger before onset of labor.

Formation of Bag of Forewater

It bulges through the cervix and becomes tense during uterine contractions.

First Stage of Labor

History

Past Obstetric History in detailes

History of Present Pregnancy

– Duration of pregnancy.

– Review of the patient's prenatal care.

– Medical disorders during this pregnancy.

– Complications during this pregnancy as antepartum hemorrhage.

History of Present Labor

– Labor pains: onset, frequency and duration.

– Passage of "show", fluid or blood per vaginum.

– Sensation of fetal movement.

Examination

General Examination

– Height and built.

– Maternal vital signs: pulse, temperature and blood pressure.

– Chest and heart examination.

– Lower limbs for oedema.

Abdominal Examination (Leopold Maneuvers)

– Fundal grip

The initial maneuver involves the examiner placing both hands on each upper quadrant of the patient's abdomen and gently palpating the fundus.

If it is the fetus' head, it should feel hard and round.

In a breech presentation, a large, nodular body is felt.

– Umbilical grip

The second maneuver involves palpation in the paraumbilical regions with both hands by applying gentle but deep pressure.

The purpose is to differentiate fetal spine (a hard, resistant structure) from its limbs (irregular, mobile small parts) to determinate the fetus' position.

- First pelvic grip

The third maneuver is suprapubic palpation by using the thumb and fingers of the dominant hand.

As with the first maneuver, the examiner ascertains the fetus' presentation and estimates its station.

If the presenting part is not engaged, a movable body (usually the fetal occiput) can be felt.

- Second pelvic grip

The fourth maneuver involves palpation of bilateral lower quadrants with the examiner stands facing the mother's feet.

The aim is to determine if the presenting part of the fetus is engaged in the mother's pelvis.

With the tips of the first 3 fingers of both hands, the examiner exerts deep pressure in the direction of the axis of the pelvic inlet.

In a cephalic presentation, the fetus' head is considered engaged if the examiner's hands diverge as they trace the head into the pelvis.

- Fundal level

- FHS

- Scar of previous operations (e.g. C.S., myomectomy)

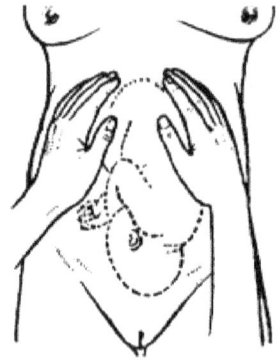

(1) Fundal Grip

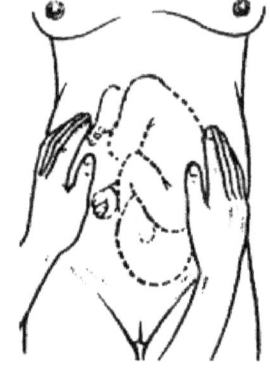

(2) Umbilical Grip

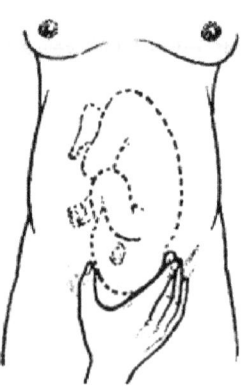

(3) First Pelvic Grip

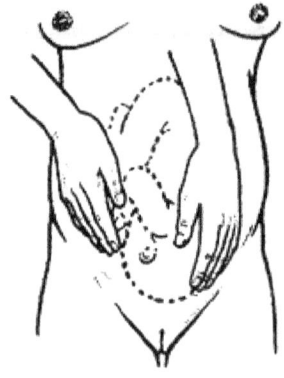

(4) Second Pelvic Grip

Abdominal Examination (Leopold Maneuvers)

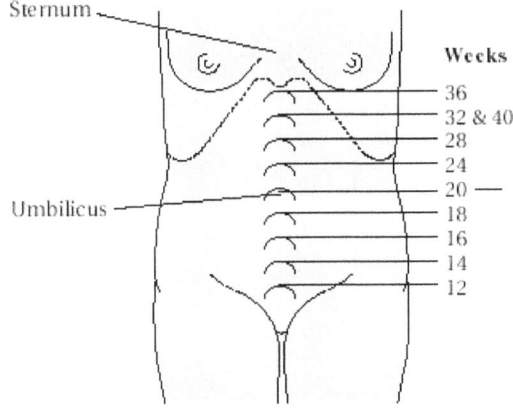

Fundal Level

Pelvic Examination

Pelvic examination is often performed using sterile gloves to decrease the risk of infection.

If membrane rupture is suspected, examination with a sterile speculum is performed to confirm pooling of amniotic fluid in the posterior fornix.

The examiner also looks for fern on a dried sample of the vaginal fluid under a microscope and checks the pH of the fluid by using a nitrazine stick or litmus paper, which turns blue if the amniotic fluid is alkalotic.

If frank bleeding is present, pelvic examination should be deferred until placenta previa is excluded with ultrasonography.

Furthermore, the pattern of contraction and the patient's presenting history may provide clues about placental abruption.

Digital examination of the cervix determines the following:

– Cervical dilatation, which ranges from 0 cm (closed or fingertip) to 10 cm (complete or fully dilated).

– Cervical effacement (assessment of the cervical length).

– Cervical position (anterior or posterior).

– Cervical consistency (soft or firm).

Palpation of the presenting part of the fetus allows the examiner to establish its station, by quantifying the distance of the body (-5 to +5 cm) that is presenting relative to the maternal ischial spines, where 0 station is in line with the plane of the maternal ischial spines).

The pelvic planes include the following:

– Pelvic inlet

The obstetrical conjugate is the distance between the sacral promontory and the inner pubic arch; it should measure 11.5 cm or more.

The diagonal conjugate is the distance from the undersurface of the pubic arch to sacral promontory.

It is 2 cm longer than the obstetrical conjugate.

The transverse diameter of the pelvic inlet measures 13.5 cm.

– Midpelvis

The midpelvis is the distance between the bony points of ischial spines, and it typically exceeds 12 cm.

- Pelvic outlet

The pelvic outlet is the distance between the ischial tuberosities and the pubic arch, and usually exceeds 10 cm.

The shape of the mother's pelvis can also be assessed and classified into 4 broad categories: gynecoid, anthropoid, android, and platypelloid.

Although the gynecoid and anthropoid pelvic shapes are thought to be most favorable for vaginal delivery, many women can be classified into 1 or more pelvic types, and such distinctions can be arbitrary.

Investigations

If not done before or if indicated:

- Complete blood cell (CBC) count.

- Blood group, Rh typing.

- Urine for albumin and sugar.

- Ultrasonography.

Workup

Evacuation of the Rectum

By enema to:

- Avoid uterine inertia.

- Help the descent of the presenting part.

- Avoid contamination by faeces during delivery.

Evacuation of the Bladder

Ask the patient to micturate every 2-3 hours.

If she can not, use a catheter.

It prevents uterine inertia.

It also helps descent of the presenting part.

Preparation of the Vulva

Shave the vulva, and clean it with soap and warm water from above downwards.

Swab it with antiseptic lotion, and apply a sterile pad.

Nutrition

When labor is established no oral feeding is allowed, but sips of water.

If labor is delayed more than 8 hours, IV drip of glucose 5% or saline-glucose solution is given.

Posture

Patient is allowed to walk during the early first stage particularly with intact membranes.

If rest is needed the patient lies on her left lateral position to prevent inferior vena cava compression and hence placental insufficiency.

Patient should not bear down during the first stage as this is useless, exhausts the patient and predisposes to genital prolapse.

Pain Control

Ideal pain releif should: provide good analgesia, and be safe for the mother and fetus, and in the same time reversible if necessary

Agents given in intermittent doses for systemic pain control include the following:

– Meperidine, 25-50 mg IV / 1-2 hours or 50-100 mg IM / 2-4 hours.

– Fentanyl, 50-100 mcg IV / hour.

– Nalbuphine, 10 mg IV or IM / 3 hours.

– Butorphanol, 1-2 mg IV or IM / 4 hours.

– Morphine, 2-5 mg IV or 10 mg IM / 4 hours.

As an alternative, regional anesthesia may be given including the following:

– Epidural

It provides the most effective pain relief.

A plastic catheter is introduced into the epidural space through a needle with a curved tip.

Intermittent doses of a local anaesthetic are injected through the catheter.

– Spinal

– Combined spinal-epidural

The Partogram

The frequency and strength of uterine contractions and changes in cervix and in the fetus' station and position should be assessed periodically to evaluate the progression of labor.

Although progression must be monitored, vaginal examinations should be performed only when necessary to minimize the risk of chorioamnionitis, particularly in women whose amniotic membrane has ruptured.

Partogram is the graphic recording of the course of labor including the following observations:

– Pulse every 30 minutes.

– Blood pressure every 2 hours.

– Temperature every 4 hours.

– Uterine contractions: frequency, strength and duration every 30 minutes by manual palpation or better by tocography if available.

– FHR monitoring every 15 minutes, particularly during and immediately after uterine contractions.

– Cervical dilatation.

– Descent of the presenting part.

– Degree of moulding.

– Fluid input and output.

– Drugs including oxytocins.

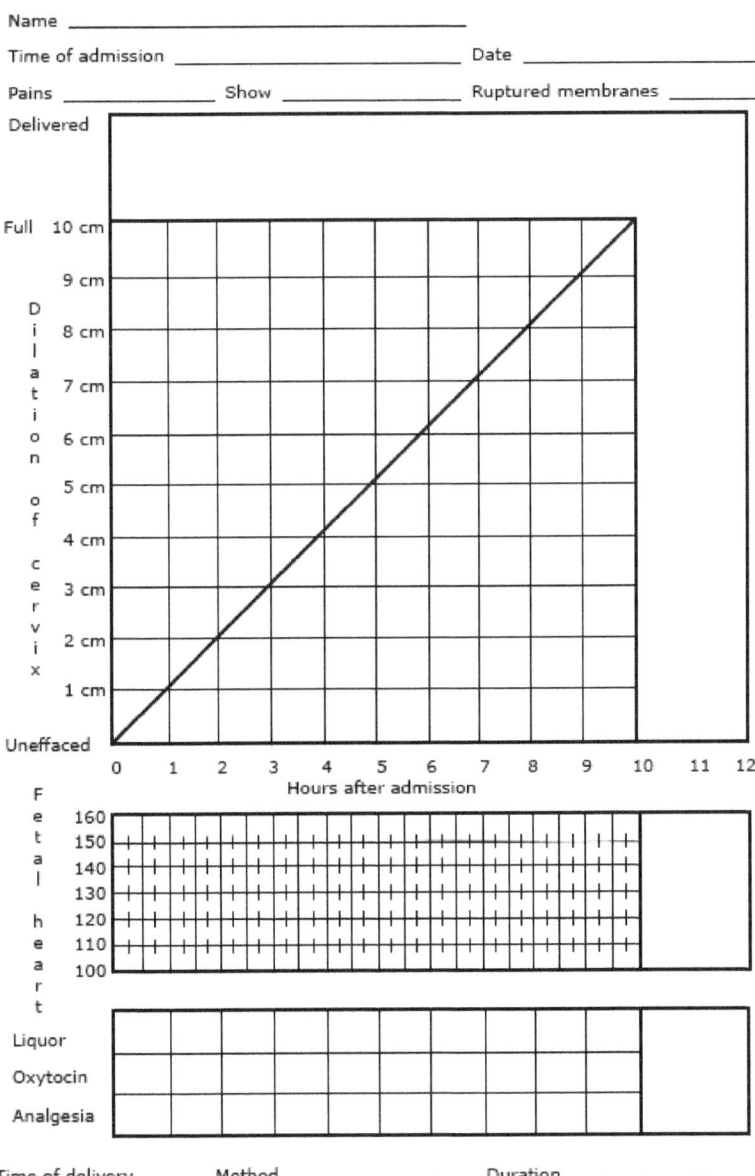

Name _____

Time of admission _____ Date _____

Pains _____ Show _____ Ruptured membranes _____

Partogram

Cardiotocography (CTG)

Is more valuable for continuous monitoring of both uterine contractions and FHR particularly in high risk pregnancy.

Cardiotography as a form of fetal assessment in labor was reviewed using randomized and quasirandomized controlled trials involving a comparison of continuous cardiotocography with no monitoring, intermittent auscultation, or intermittent cardiotocography.

This review concluded that continuous cardiotocography during labor is associated with a reduction in neonatal seizures but not cerebral palsy or infant mortality; however, continuous monitoring is associated with increased cesarean and operative vaginal deliveries.

If nonreassuring fetal heart rate tracings by cardiotography (eg, late decelerations) are noted, a fetal scalp electrode may be applied to generate sensitive readings of beat-to-beat variability.

However, a fetal scalp electrode should be avoided if the mother has HIV, hepatitis B or hepatitis C infections, or if fetal thrombocytopenia is suspected.

A framework has been suggested to classify and standardize the interpretation of a fetal heart rate monitoring pattern according to the risk of fetal acidemia with the intention of minimizing neonatal acidemia without excessive obstetric intervention.

The existing data provide limited support for the use of fetal pulse oximetry when used in the presence of a nonreassuring fetal heart rate tracing to reduce cesarean delivery for nonreassuring fetal status.

Further evaluation of a fetus at risk for labor intolerance or distress can be accomplished with blood sampling from fetal scalp capillaries.

This procedure allows for a direct assessment of fetal oxygenation and blood pH.

A pH of < 7.20 warrants further investigation for the fetus' well-being and for possible resuscitation or surgical intervention.

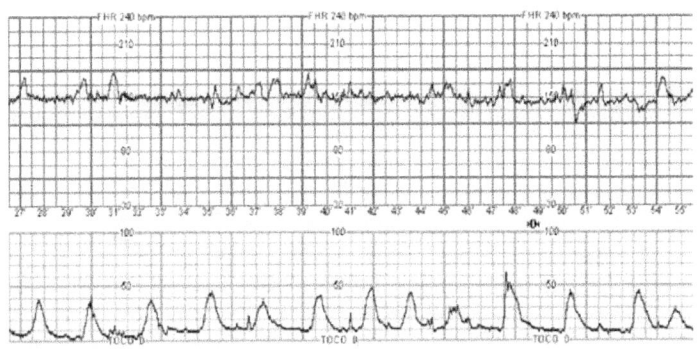

Cardiotocography (CTG)

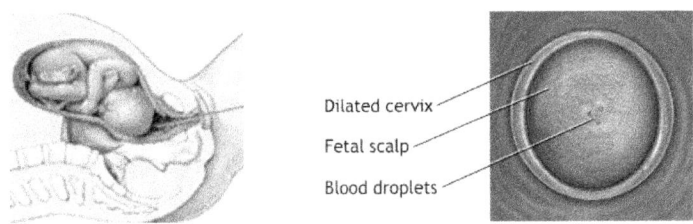

Dilated cervix

Fetal scalp

Blood droplets

Fetal Scalp pH Testing

Augmention of Labor

Two methods of augmenting labor have been established.

The traditional method involves the use of low doses of oxytocin with long intervals between dose increments.

For example, low-dose infusion of oxytocin is started at 1 mili IU/min and increased by 1-2 mili IU/min every 20-30 minutes until adequate uterine contraction is obtained.

The second method, or active management of labor, involves a protocol of clinical management that aims to optimize uterine contractions and shorten labor.

This protocol includes strict criteria for admission to the labor and delivery unit, early amniotomy, hourly cervical examinations, early diagnosis of inefficient uterine activity (if the cervical dilation rate is < 1.0 cm/h), and high-dose oxytocin infusion if uterine activity is inefficient.

Oxytocin infusion starts at 4 mili IU/min (or even 6 mili IU/min) and increases by 4 mili IU/min (or 6 mili IU/min) every 15 minutes until a rate of 7 contractions per 15 minutes is achieved or until the maximum infusion rate of 36 mili IU/min is reached.

Data from randomized controlled trials confirmed that active management of labor shortens the first stage of labor and reduces the likelihood of maternal febrile morbidity, but it does not consistently decrease the probability of cesarean delivery, and a number of risk factors are associated with a failure of labor to progress.

These risk factors include premature rupture of the membranes (PROM), nulliparity, induction of labor, increasing maternal age, and or other complications (eg, previous perinatal death, pregestational or gestational diabetes mellitus, hypertension, infertility treatment).

While the ACOG defines labor dystocia as abnormal labor that results form abnormalities of the power (uterine contractions or maternal expulsive forces), the passenger (position, size, or presentation of the fetus), or the passage (pelvis or soft tissues), labor dystocia can rarely be diagnosed with certainty.

Often, a "failure to progress" in the first stage is diagnosed if uterine contraction pattern exceeds 200 Montevideo units for 2 hours without cervical change during the active phase of labor is encountered.

Thus, the traditional criteria to diagnose active-phase arrest are cervical dilatation of at least 4 cm, cervical changes of < 1 cm in 2 hours, and a uterine contraction pattern of > 200 Montevideo units.

These findings are also a common indication for cesarean delivery.

This protocol achieved vaginal delivery rates of 56-61% in nulliparas and 88% in multiparas without severe adverse maternal or neonatal outcomes.

SECOND STAGE OF LABOR

It is the stage of expulsion of the fetus.

Begins with full cervical dilatation.

Ends with the delivery of the fetus.

Its duration is about 1 hour in primigravida and 30 minutes in multipara.

MECHANISM

The ability of the fetus to successfully negotiate the pelvis during labor involves changes in position of its head during its passage in labor.

The mechanisms of labor, also known as the cardinal movements, are described in relation to a vertex presentation, as is the case in 95% of all pregnancies.

Although labor and delivery occurs in a continuous fashion, the cardinal movements of labor are described as discrete sequences, as discussed below.

Engagement

The widest diameter of the presenting part (with a well-flexed head, where the largest transverse diameter of the fetal occiput is the biparietal diameter) enters the maternal pelvis in the oblique or transverse diameter of the pelvic inlet.

On the pelvic examination, the presenting part is at 0 station, or at the level of the maternal ischial spines.

Descent

The downward passage of the presenting part through the pelvis.

It is continuous throughout labor particularly during the second stage and caused by:

- Uterine contractions and retractions.

- The auxiliary forces which is bearing down brought by contraction of the diaphragm and abdominal muscles.

- The unfolding of the fetus i.e. straightening of its body due to contractions of the circular muscles of the uterus.

Flexion

As the fetal vertex descents, it encounters resistance from the bony pelvis or the soft tissues of the pelvic floor, resulting in passive flexion of the fetal occiput.

The suboccipito-bregmatic diameter (9.5 cm) passes through the birth canal instead of the suboccipito-frontal diameter (10 cm).

Internal Rotation

As the head descends, the occiputis rotated about 45° in the direction of levator ani muscles i.e. downwards, forwards and inwards.

It occurs at the level of the plane of the greatest pelvic dimension.

Internal rotation brings the anteroposterior diameter of the head in line with the anteroposterior diameter of the pelvic outlet.

Extension

With further descent and full flexion of the head, the base of the occiput comes in contact with the inferior margin of the pubic symphysis.

Upward resistance from the pelvic floor and downward forces from the uterine contractions cause the occiput to extend around the symphysis.

This is followed by the delivery of the fetus' head.

Restitution

When the fetus' head is free of resistance, it untwists about 45° left or right, returning to its original anatomic position in relation to the body (undo the twist of the neck caused by internal rotation).

External Rotation

The shoulders enter the pelvis in the opposite oblique diameter to that previously passed by the head.

When the anterior shoulder meets the pelvic floor it rotates anteriorly 45°.

This movement is transmitted to the head so it rotates 45° in the same direction of restitution.

Expulsion

After the fetus' head is delivered, further descent brings the anterior shoulder to the level of the pubic symphysis.

The posterior shoulder is delivered first by lateral flexion of the spine.

The anterior shoulder then follows, then the rest of the body.

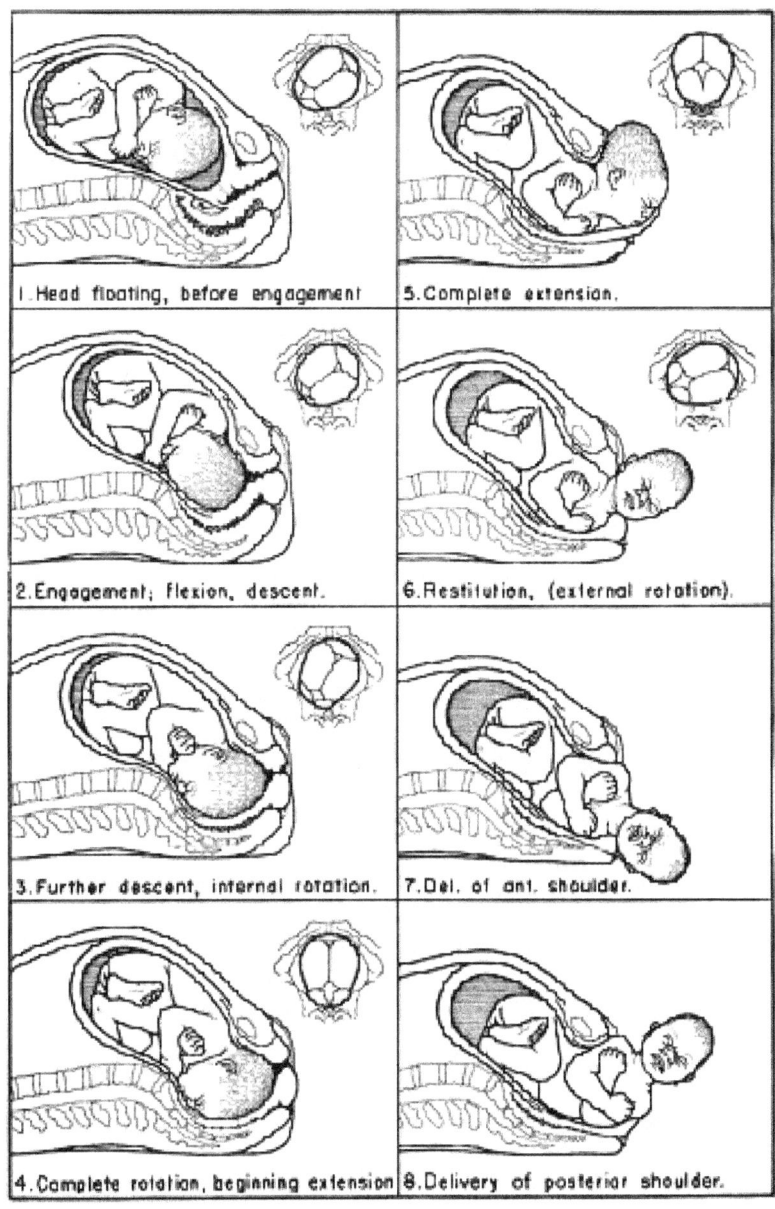

1. Head floating, before engagement
2. Engagement; flexion, descent.
3. Further descent, internal rotation.
4. Complete rotation, beginning extension
5. Complete extension.
6. Restitution, (external rotation).
7. Del. of ant. shoulder.
8. Delivery of posterior shoulder.

Cardinal Movements of Labor

MANAGEMENT

When the woman enters the second stage of labor with complete cervical dilatation, the fetal heart rate should be monitored or auscultated at least every 5 minutes and after each contraction during the second stage.

Although the parturient may be encouraged to push in concordance with the contractions during the second stage, many women with epidural anesthesia who do not feel the urge to push may allow the fetus to descend passively, with a period of rest before active pushing begins.

A number of randomized controlled trials have shown that, in nulliparous women, delayed pushing, or passive descend, is not associated with adverse perinatal outcomes or an increased risk for operative deliveries despite an often prolonged second stage of labor.

When a prolonged second stage of labor is encountered, clinical assessment of the parturient, the fetus, and the expulsive forces is warranted.

A randomized controlled trial determined that application of fundal pressure on the uterus does not shorten the second stage of labor.

Although the 2003 ACOG practice guidelines state that the duration of the second stage alone does not mandate intervention by operative vaginal delivery or cesarean delivery if progress is being made, the clinician has several management options (continuing observation / expectant management, operative vaginal delivery by forceps or vacuum-assisted vaginal delivery, or cesarean delivery) when second-stage arrest is diagnosed.

Delivery of the Fetus

When delivery is imminent, the mother is usually positioned supine with her knees bent (ie, dorsal lithotomy position), though delivery can occur with the mother in any position, including the lateral (Sims) position, the partial sitting or squatting position, or on her hands and knees.

The lower abdomen, upper parts of the thighs, vulva and perineum are swabbed with antiseptic lotion.

Sterile legs and towels are applied.

Ask the patient to bear down during contractions and relax in between.

Although an episiotomy used to be routinely performed at this time, the ACOG recommended in 2006 that its use be restricted to maternal or fetal indications.

Mediolateral

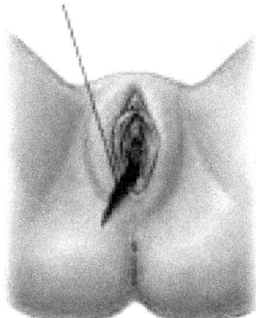

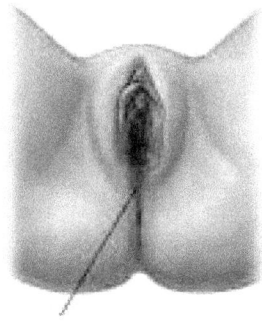

Midline

Episiotomy

Delivery of the Head

Crowning is the word used to describe when the fetal head forcibly extends the vaginal outlet.

Ritgen maneuver can be performed to deliver the head.

Draped with a sterile towel, the heel of the clinician's hand is placed over the posterior perineum overlying the fetal chin, and pressure is applied upward to extend the fetus' head.

The other hand is placed over the fetus' occiput, with pressure applied downward to flex its head.

Thus, the head is held in mid position until it is delivered, followed by suctioning of the oropharynx and nares.

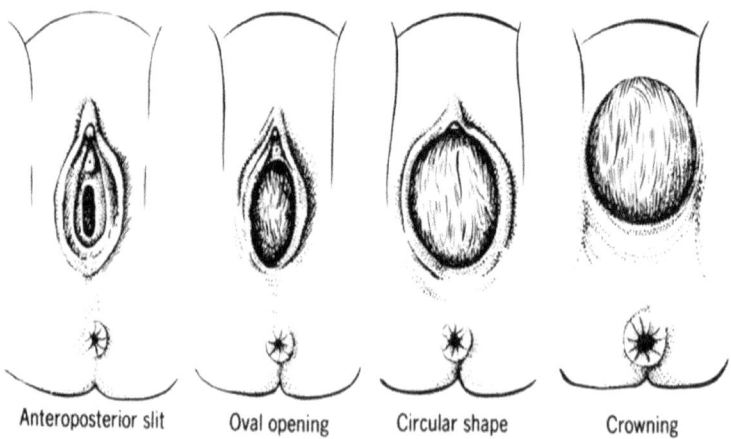

Anteroposterior slit   Oval opening   Circular shape   Crowning

Crowning

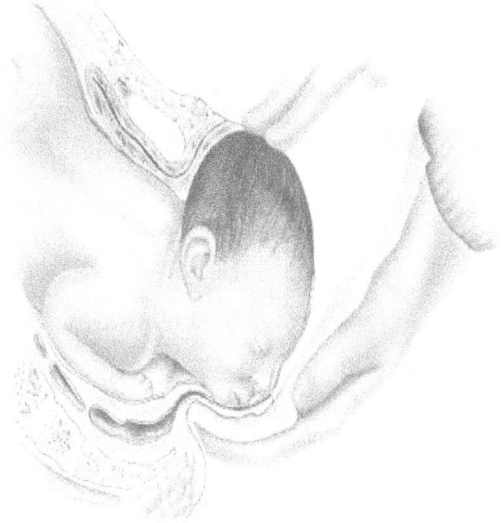

Ritgen Maneuver

Delivery of the Shoulders

Gentle downward traction is applied to the head till the anterior shoulder slips under the symphysis pubis.

The head is lifted upwards to deliver the posterior shoulder first then downwards to deliver the anterior shoulder.

Of note, some providers, in an attempt to avoid shoulder dystocia, deliver the anterior shoulder prior to restitution of the fetal head.

Delivery of the Body

Usually slips without difficulty otherwise gentle traction is applied to complete delivery.

Clamping the Cord

The baby is held by its ankles with the head downwards at a lower level than its mother for few seconds.

This is contraindicated in preterm babies, erythroblastosis fetalis, and suspicion of intracranial hemorrhage.

This may be enhanced by milking the cord towards the baby, to add about 100 ml of blood to its circulation.

The cord is divided between 2 clamps to avoid bleeding from a possible second uniovular twin.

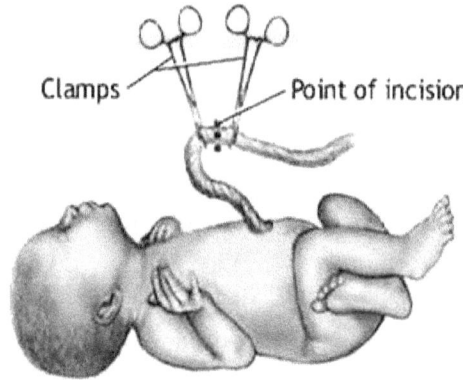

Clamping the Cord

THIRD STAGE OF LABOR

It is the stage of expulsion of the placenta and membranes.

Begins after delivery of the fetus.

Ends with expulsion of the placenta and membranes.

Its duration is about 10-20 minutes in both primi and multipara.

MECHANISM

The third stage is composed of 3 phases: placental separation, descent, and expulsion.

After delivery of the fetus, the uterus continues to contract and retract.

As the placenta is inelastic, it starts to separate through the spongiosa layer by one of the following mechanisms:

Schultze's Mechanism (80%)

The central area of the placenta separates first and placenta is delivered like an inverted umbrella.

There is less blood loss and less liability for retention of fragments.

Duncan's Mechanism (20%)

The lower edge of the placenta separates first and placenta is delivered side ways.

There is more liability of bleeding and retained fragments.

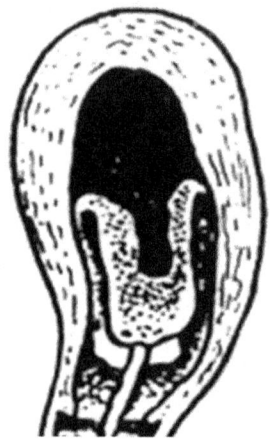

Schultze's Mechanism

Duncan's Mechanism

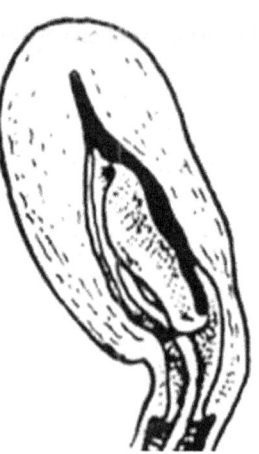

Mechanism of Placental Delivery

MANAGEMENT

Delivery of Placenta

Conservative (Expectant) Method

Put the ulnar border of the left hand just above the fundus at the level of the umbilicus to detect any bleeding inside the uterus known by rising level of the atonic uterus.

Wait for signs of placental separation and descent but do not massage the uterus.

<u>Signs of Placental Separation and Descent</u>

- The body of the uterus becomes smaller, harder and globular.

- The fundal level rises as the upper segment overrides the lower uterine segment which is now distended with the placenta.

- Suprapubic bulge due to presence of the placenta in the lower uterine segment.

- Elongation of the cord particularly on pressing on the uterine fundus and it does not recede back into the vagina on relieving the pressure.

- Gush of blood from the vagina.

As soon as these signs are detected massage the uterus to induce its contraction.

Ask the patient to bear down and push the uterus downwards to deliver the placenta.

Hold the placenta between the two hands and roll it to make the membranes like a rope in order not to miss a part of it.

Give ergometrine 0.5 mg or oxytocin 5 units IM after delivery of the placenta to help uterine contraction and minimise blood loss.

These may be given before delivery of the placenta.

Active (Brandt-Andrews) Method

With delivery of the anterior shoulder, 0.5 mg ergometrine or syntometrine (0.5 mg ergometrine + 5 units oxytocin) is given IM.

When the uterus contracts, put the left hand suprapubic and push the uterus upwards while gentle downward and backward traction is applied on the cord by the right hand.

When the placenta is delivered it is rolled as in the conservative method.

A review of 5 randomized trials comparing active versus expectant management of the third stage demonstrated that active management was associated with lowered risks of maternal blood loss, postpartum hemorrhage, and prolongation of the third stage, but it increased maternal nausea, vomiting, and blood pressure (when ergometrine was used).

However, given the reduced risk of complications, this review recommends that active management is superior to expectant management and should be the routine management of choice.

Therefore, if the risks and benefits are balanced, active management with oxytocin may be considered apart of routine management of the third stage.

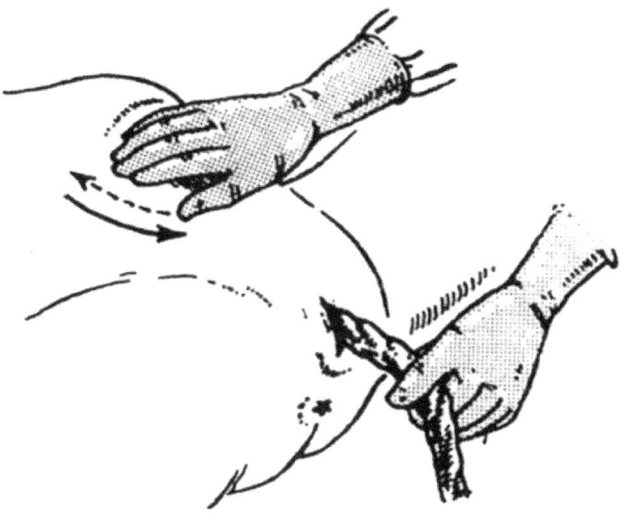

Brandt-Andrews Method

After Delivery of Placenta

Examine the placenta and membranes by exploring it on a plain surface to be sure that it is complete.

If there is missed part, exploration of the uterus is done under general anaesthesia.

Ongoing blood loss and a boggy uterus suggest uterine atony.

A thorough examination of the birth canal, including the cervix and the vagina, the perineum, and the distal rectum, is warranted, and repair of episiotomy or perineal / vaginal lacerations should be carried out.

Care of the Newborn

Clearance of Air Passages

The newborn is placed in supine position with the head lower down.

A metal, rubber or better disposable plastic catheter is used to aspirate the mucus from the pharynx and mouth directly by the physician's mouth or by attach it to an electric suction pump.

Crying of the baby is usually occurs within seconds, if delayed slapping its soles, flexion and extension of the legs and rubbing the back usually stimulate breathing.

Apgar Score

Is calculated at 1 and 5 minutes and further steps of resuscitation are arranged according to it.

Umbilical Cord

A disposable plastic umbilical clamp is applied about 5 cm from the umbilicus to avoid the possibility of tying an umbilical hernia then cut about 1.5 cm distal to the clamp.

Inspect for bleeding and paint it with alcohol.

Weight

Weight the newborn and record it.

Congenital Anomalies

The newborn is examined for injuries or congenital anomalies.

Care of Eyes

An antibiotic eye drops are instilled into the eyes as a prophylaxis against ophthalmia neonatorum.

Dressing

Dressing as well as all previous procedures should be done in a warm place better under radiant warmer to prevent heat loss which occurs rapidly after delivery increasing the metabolism and acidosis.

Identification

Identification of the baby by a plastic bracelet on which its mother's name is written.

Fourth Stage of Labor

It is the stage of early recovery.

Begins immediately after expulsion of the placenta and membranes.

Lasts for one hour.

Routine uterine massage is usually done every 15 minutes during this period.

Careful observation for the patient, particularly atony of the uterus and vaginal bleeding is essential.

ABNORMAL LABOR

To define abnormal labor, a definition of normal labor must be understood and accepted.

By following thousands of labors resulting in uncomplicated vaginal deliveries, time limits and progress milestones have been identified that define normal labor.

Failure to meet these milestones defines abnormal labor, which suggests an increased risk of an unfavorable outcome.

Thus, abnormal labor alerts alternative methods for a successful delivery that minimize risks to both the mother and the infant.

Dystocia of labor is defined as difficult labor or abnormally slow progress of labor.

Other terms that are often used interchangeably with dystocia are dysfunctional labor, failure to progress (lack of progressive cervical dilatation or lack of descent), and cephalopelvic disproportion.

Friedman's 1955 defined the following three stages of labor:

– The first stage starts with uterine contractions leading to complete cervical dilation and is divided into latent and active phases.

– The second stage of labor is defined as complete dilation of the cervix to the delivery of the infant.

– The third stage of labor involves delivery of the placenta.

Abnormal Labor Indicators

Indication	Nullipara	Multipara
Prolonged latent phase	>20 h	>14 h
Average second stage	50 min	20 min
Prolonged second stage	>2 h	>1 h
Protracted dilation	<1.2 cm/h	<1.5 cm/h
Protracted descent	<1 cm/h	<2 cm/h
Arrest of dilation	>2 h	>2 h
Arrest of descent	>2 h	>1 h
Prolonged third stage	>30 min	>30 min

Abnormal labor constitutes any findings that fall outside the accepted normal labor curve.

However, the authors hesitate to apply the diagnosis of abnormal labor during the latent phase because it is easy to confuse prodromal contractions for latent labor.

For both nulliparous and multiparous women, labor may take longer than 6 hours to progress from 4 cm to 5 cm and longer than 3 hours to progress from 5 cm to 6 cm of dilation.

Cervical dilation of 6 cm appears to be a better landmark for the start of the active phase.

The 95th percentile for duration of the second stage in a nulliparous woman with conduction anesthesia is closer to 4 hours.

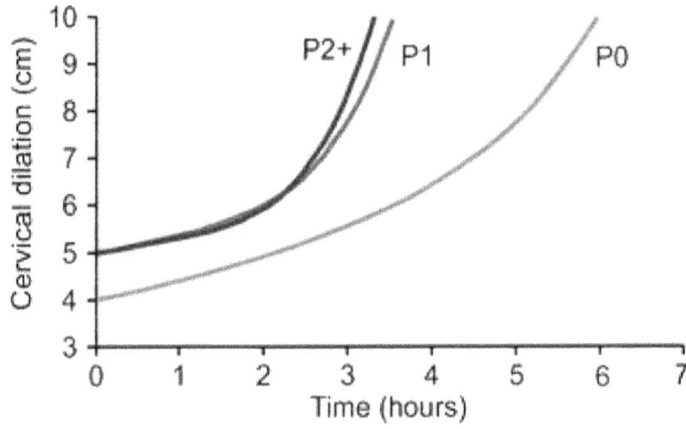

Labor Curves by Parity

First Stage of Labor

Diagnosis of abnormal labor during the latent phase is uncommon and likely an incorrect diagnosis.

Around the time uterine contractions cause the cervix to become 3-4 cm, the patient usually enters the active phase of the first stage of labor.

Both ACOG and the Consortium on Safe Labor have proposed extending the minimum period before diagnosing active-phase arrest.

The Consortium on Safe Labor defines 6 hours as the 95th percentile of time to go from 4 cm to 5 cm dilation, with the active phase defined as beginning at 6 cm (instead of 4 cm).

The ACOG has also stated that extending the time from 2 to 4 hours with oxytocin augmentation appears effective.

Irrespective of the duration, maternal and fetal well-being status must be confirmed.

The maternal risk of a first stage greater than the 95th percentile (>30 h) is associated with a higher cesarean delivery rate and chorioamnionitis.

The neonatal risk is associated with a higher incidence of neonatal ICU admissions in the absence of any other of the major morbidities.

Second Stage of Labor

The Consortium on Safe Labor also addressed the 95th percentile for the second stage for nulliparous women; it was 2.8 hours (168 min) without regional anesthesia and 3.6 hours (216 min) with regional anesthesia.

For multiparous women, the 95th percentiles for second-stage duration with and without regional anesthesia remained around 2 hours and 1 hour, respectively.

However, other studies demonstrate the risks of both maternal and perinatal adverse outcomes rising with increased duration of the second stage, particularly for durations longer than 3 hours in nulliparous women and 2 hours in multiparous women.

Thus, careful clinical assessment of fetal and maternal well-being must be confirmed when extending the duration of the first and second stages of labor.

A prolonged latent phase may result from oversedation or from entering labor early with a thickened or uneffaced cervix.

It may be misdiagnosed in the face of frequent prodromal contractions.

Protraction of active labor is more easily diagnosed and is dependent upon the 3 *P*'s.

The first *P,* the passenger, may produce abnormal labor because of the infant's size (eg, macrosomia) or from malpresentation.

The second *P,* the pelvis, can cause abnormal labor because its contours may be too small or narrow to allow passage of the infant.

Both the passenger and pelvis cause abnormal labor by a mechanical obstruction, referred to as mechanical dystocia.

With the third *P,* the power component, the frequency of uterine contraction may be adequate, but the intensity may be inadequate.

Disruption of communication between adjacent segments of the uterus may also exist, resulting from surgical scarring, fibroids, or other.

Whatever the cause, the contraction pattern fails to result in cervical effacement and dilation; this is called functional dystocia.

Evaluation

Evaluate every pregnant patient who presents with contractions in the labor and delivery unit.

Any patient in labor is at risk for abnormal labor regardless of the number of previous pregnancies or adequate dimensions of the pelvis.

Plot the progress of any patient in labor, and evaluate it on a labor curve.

Upon admission to the labor and delivery unit, determine and document clinical findings.

Clinical pelvimetry, which is best performed at the first prenatal care visit, is important in order to assess the pelvic type (eg, android, gynecoid, platypelloid, anthropoid).

Evaluate the position of the fetal head in early labor because caput and moulding complicate correct assessment as labor progresses.

Establish and document an estimated fetal weight.

Monitor fetal heart rate and uterine contraction patterns to assess fetal well-being and adequacy of labor.

Perform a cervical examination to determine whether the patient is in the latent or active phase of labor.

Addressing these issues allows for an assessment of the current phase of labor and anticipation of whether abnormal labor from any of the 3 *P*'s may be encountered.

Management

A prolonged latent phase is not indicative of dystocia in itself because this diagnosis cannot be made in the latent phase.

For those in the latent phase, the treatment of choice is rest for several hours, and uterine activity, fetal status, and cervical effacement must be evaluated to determine if progress to the active phase has occurred.

Approximately 85% of patients so treated progress to the active phase.

Approximately 10% will cease to have contractions, and the diagnosis of false labor may be made.

For the approximately 5% of patients in whom therapeutic rest fails and in patients for whom expeditious delivery is indicated, oxytocin infusion may be used.

Anecdotal reports have stated that simply repositioning the patient frequently relieves a seemingly obstructed labor.

In theory, it may unseat an asynclitic or malrotated presenting part and allow it to engage in the pelvis more effectively.

Induction of Labor

In a large cohort of nulliparous women who delivered singleton live births at 39-42 weeks, induction of labor was not associated with an increased risk of cesarean delivery compared with delivery at a later gestational age.

Additionally, the risk of labor dystocia for women who were induced at 39 weeks (5.93%) was lower than for those expectantly managed.

Labor dystocia was also less likely for women who had induction at 40 weeks compared with delivery later.

Additionally, no difference in risk of operative vaginal delivery, including forceps or vacuum-assisted vaginal delivery, was reported.

While these data support that induction may provide improved perinatal outcomes, without impacting labor dystocia or increasing cesarean delivery rate, the authors caution generalized implementation and recommend future large prospective, randomized, clinical trials to further assess the potential benefit in low-risk populations.

Probably the most common complication of the medical induction of labor is hyperstimulation of the uterus.

If untreated, excessive stimulation of the uterus can result in fetal compromise, cord compression, and uteroplacental insufficiency.

Uterine rupture, postpartum uterine atony, and postpartum hemorrhage may occur and can be life-threatening complications.

Amniotomy

Amniotomy is often used and has become an accepted practice once the patient has reached the active phase of labor, although it has not been shown to result in shorter labor.

This practice is not recommended in the latent phase because it may only serve to increase the risk of intrauterine infection or cord prolapse.

Vaginal / Cesarean Delivery

If one of the arrest or protraction disorders is identified and fails to respond to conservative measures, or if the fetal heart pattern is nonreassuring, expedient delivery is justified.

This includes operative vaginal delivery (if appropriate) or cesarean delivery as indicated.

REFERENCES

– Aasheim V, Nilsen A, Lukasse M, et al. Perineal techniques during the second stage of labour for reducing perineal trauma. Cochrane Database Syst Rev. 2011; 12: CD006672.

– ACOG. American College of Obstetricians and Gynecologists Practice Bulletin. Obstetric Analgesia and Anesthesia. Clinical Management Guidelines for Obstetricians-Gynecologists. No 36. American College of Obstetricians and Gynecologists: Washington, DC; 2002.

– ACOG. American College of Obstetricians and Gynecologists Practice Bulletin. Dystocia and augmentation of labor. Clinical management guidelines for Obstetricians-Gynecologists. No 49. American College of Obstetricians and Gynecologists: Washington, DC; 2003.

– ACOG. American College of Obstetricians and Gynecologists Practice Bulletin. Intrapartum Fetal Heart Rate Monitoring. Clinical Management Guidelines for Obstetricians-Gynecologists. No 36. American College of Obstetricians and Gynecologists: Washington, DC; 2005.

– ACOG. American College of Obstetricians and Gynecologists Practice Bulletin. Episiotomy. Clinical Management Guidelines for Obstetricians-Gynecologists. No 71. American College of Obstetricians and Gynecologists: Washington, DC; 2006.

– ACOG Practice Bulletin No. 80: premature rupture of membranes. Clinical management guidelines for obstetrician-gynecologists. Obstet Gynecol. 2007; 109: 1007-19.

– Albers L, Schiff M, Gorwoda J. The length of active labor in normal pregnancies. Obstet Gynecol. 1996; 87: 355-9.

– Alexander J, Sharma S, McIntire D, et al. Epidural analgesia lengthens the Friedman active phase of labor. Obstet Gynecol. 2002; 100: 46-50.

– Alfirevic Z, Devane D, Gyte G. Continuous cardiotocography (CTG) as a form of electronic fetal monitoring (EFM) for fetal assessment during labour. Cochrane Database Syst Rev. 2006; 3: CD006066.

– Allen V, Baskett T, O'Connell C, et al. Maternal and perinatal outcomes with increasing duration of the second stage of labor. Obstet Gynecol. 2009; 113: 1248-58.

– Andersson O, Hellstrom-Westas L, Andersson D, et al. Effect of delayed versus early umbilical cord clamping on neonatal outcomes and iron status at 4 months: a randomised controlled trial. BMJ. 2011; 343: d7157.

– Api O, Balcin M, Ugurel V, et al. The effect of uterine fundal pressure on the duration of the second stage of labor: a randomized controlled trial. Acta Obstet Gynecol Scand. 2009; 88: 320-4.

– Beckmann C, Ling F, Barzansky BM. Obstetrics and Gynecology. 4th ed. Philadelphia, Pa: Lippincott Williams & Wilkins; 2001.

– Bloom S, McIntire D, Kelly M, et al. Lack of effect of walking on labor and delivery. N Engl J Med. 1998; 339: 76-9.

– Bloom S, Casey B, Schaffer J, et al. A randomized trial of coached versus uncoached maternal pushing during the second stage of labor. Am J Obstet Gynecol. 2006; 194: 10-3.

– Bofill J, Rust O, Perry K, et al. Forceps and vacuum delivery: a survey of North American residency programs. Obstet Gynecol. 1996; 88: 622-5.

– Bofill J, Vincent R, Ross E, et al. Nulliparous active labor, epidural analgesia, and cesarean delivery for dystocia. Am J Obstet Gynecol. 1997; 177: 1465-70.

– Cheng Y, Hopkins L, Caughey A. How long is too long: Does a prolonged second stage of labor in nulliparous women affect maternal and neonatal outcomes? Am J Obstet Gynecol. 2004; 191: 933-8.

– Chinnock M, Robson S. Obstetric trainees' experience in vaginal breech delivery: implications for future practice. Obstet Gynecol. 2007; 110: 900-3.

– Creasy R, Resnik R, Iams J. Maternal-Fetal Medicine. In: Principles and Practice. 5th ed. Philadelphia, Pa: WB Saunders; 2004.

– Cunningham F, Gant N, Leveno K. Williams Obstetrics. 22nd ed. New York, NY: McGraw-Hill; 2005.

– East C, Chan F, Colditz P, et al. Fetal pulse oximetry for fetal assessment in labour. Cochrane Database Syst Rev. 2007; CD004075.

– El-Sayed Y. Diagnosis and management of arrest disorders: duration to wait. Semin Perinatol. 2012; 36: 374-8.

– Fitzpatrick M, Harkin R, McQuillan K, et al. A randomised clinical trial comparing the effects of delayed versus immediate pushing with epidural analgesia on mode of delivery and faecal continence. BJOG. 2002; 109: 1359-65.

– Friedman E, Sachtleben M. Dysfunctional labor. I. Prolonged latent phase in the nullipara. Obstet Gynecol. 1961; 17: 135-48.

– Friedman E, Sachtleben M. Dysfunctional labor. II. Protracted active-phase dilatation in the nullipara. Obstet Gynecol. 1961; 17: 566-78.

– Friedman E. Primigravid labor; a graphicostatistical analysis. Obstet Gynecol. 1955; 6: 567-89.

– Frigoletto F, Lieberman E, Lang J, et al. A clinical trial of active management of labor. N Engl J Med. 1995; 333: 745-50.

– Gabbe S, Niebyl J, Simpson J. Obstetrics Normal & Problem Pregnancies. 5th ed. New York: Churchill Livingstone; 2007.

– Grobman W, Simon C. Factors associated with the length of the latent phase during labor induction. Eur J Obstet Gynecol Reprod Biol. 2007; 132: 163-6.

– Gülmezoglu A, Villar J, Ngoc N, et al. WHO multicentre randomised trial of misoprostol in the management of the third stage of labour. Lancet. 2001; 358: 689-95.

– Hannah M, Ohlsson A, Farine D, et al. Induction of labor compared with expectant management for prelabor rupture of the membranes at term. TERMPROM Study Group. N Engl J Med. 1996; 334: 1005-10.

– Hansen S, Clark S, Foster J. Active pushing versus passive fetal descent in second stage of labor: a randomized controlled trial. Obstet Gynecol. 2002; 99: 29-34.

– Herman A, Zimerman A, Arieli S, et al. Down-up sequential separation of the placenta. Ultrasound Obstet Gynecol. 2002; 19: 278-81.

– Janni W, Schiessl B, Peschers U, et al. The prognostic impact of a prolonged second stage of labor on maternal and fetal outcome. Acta Obstet Gynecol Scand. 2002; 81: 214-21.

– Kilpatrick S, Laros R. Characteristics of normal labor. Obstet Gynecol. 1989; 74: 85-7.

– Lopez-Zeno J, Peaceman A, Adashek J, et al. A controlled trial of a program for the active management of labor. N Engl J Med. 1992; 326: 450-4.

– Martin J, Hamilton B, Sutton P, et al. Births: final data for 2004. Natl Vital Stat Rep. 2006; 55: 1-101.

– Menticoglou S, Manning F, Harman C, et al. Perinatal outcome in relation to second-stage duration. Am J Obstet Gynecol. 1995; 173: 906-12.

– Myles T, Santolaya J. Maternal and neonatal outcomes in patients with a prolonged second stage of labor. Obstet Gynecol. 2003; 102: 52-8.

– Norwitz E, Robinson J, Repke J. Labor and delivery. In: Gabbe SG, Niebyl JR, Simpson JL, eds. Obstetrics: Normal and problem pregnancies. 3rd ed. New York: Churchill Livingstone; 2003.

– O'Connell M, Hussain J, Maclennan F, et al. Factors associated with a prolonged second state of labour--a case-controlled study of 364 nulliparous labours. J Obstet Gynaecol. 2003; 23: 255-7.

– O'Driscoll K, Foley M, MacDonald D. Active management of labor as an alternative to cesarean section for dystocia. Obstet Gynecol. 1984; 63: 485-90.

– O'Driscoll K, Meagher D. Introduction. In: O'Driscoll K, Meagher D, eds. Active Management of Labour. 2nd ed. Eastbourne, United Kingdom: Balliere Tindall; 1986.

– Pattinson RC. Pelvimetry for fetal cephalic presentations at term. Cochrane Database Syst Rev. 2000; CD000161.

– Prendiville W, Elbourne D, McDonald S. Active versus expectant management in the third stage of labour. Cochrane Database Syst Rev. 2000; CD000007.

– Rabe H, Diaz-Rossello J, Duley L, et al. Effect of timing of umbilical cord clamping and other strategies to influence placental transfusion at preterm birth on maternal and infant outcomes. Cochrane Database Syst Rev. 2012; CD003248.

– Reveiz L, Gaitán HG, Cuervo L. Enemas during labour. Cochrane Database Syst Rev. 2013; CD000330.

– Rinehart B, Terrone D, Hudson C, et al. Lack of utility of standard labor curves in the prediction of progression during labor induction. Am J Obstet Gynecol. 2000; 182: 1520-6.

– Rouse D, Owen J, Hauth J. Active-phase labor arrest: oxytocin augmentation for at least 4 hours. Obstet Gynecol. 1999; 93: 323-8.

– Rouse D, Owen J, Hauth J. Criteria for failed labor induction: prospective evaluation of a standardized protocol. Obstet Gynecol. 2000; 96: 671-7.

– Sadler L, Davison T, McCowan L. A randomised controlled trial and meta-analysis of active management of labour. BJOG. 2000; 107: 909-15.

– Sheiner E, Levy A, Feinstein U, et al. Obstetric risk factors for failure to progress in the first versus the second stage of labor. J Matern Fetal Neonatal Med. 2002; 11: 409-13.

– Sheiner E, Levy A, Feinstein U, et al. Risk factors and outcome of failure to progress during the first stage of labor: a population-based study. Acta Obstet Gynecol Scand. 2002; 81: 222-6.

– Singata M, Tranmer J, Gyte G. Restricting oral fluid and food intake during labour. Cochrane Database Syst Rev. 2013; CD003930.

– Smith C, Levett K, Collins C, et al. Relaxation techniques for pain management in labour. Cochrane Database Syst Rev. 2011; 12: CD009514.

– Smyth R, Markham C, Dowswell T. Amniotomy for shortening spontaneous labour. Cochrane Database Syst Rev. 2013; CD006167.

– World Health Organization. Maternal and Child Health and Family Planning. The prevention and management of postpartum haemorrhage. Report of a technical working group. WHO/MCH. 1990.

– Zhang J, Troendle J, Yancey M. Reassessing the labor curve in nulliparous women. Am J Obstet Gynecol. 2002; 187: 824-8.

– Zhang J, Landy H, Branch D, et al. Contemporary patterns of spontaneous labor with normal neonatal outcomes. Obstet Gynecol. 2010; 116: 1281-7.

www.ingramcontent.com/pod-product-compliance
Lightning Source LLC
Chambersburg PA
CBHW070847180526
45168CB00002B/980